How to find the Bes[t] Elderly

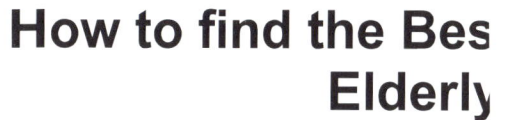

by
Jennifer King

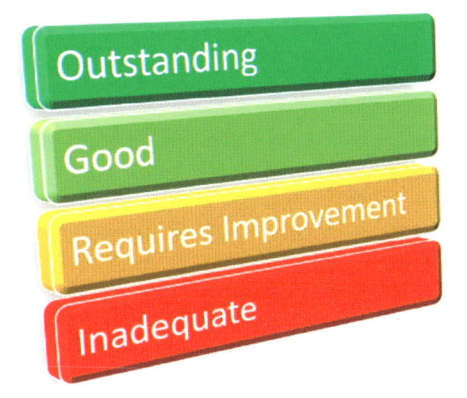

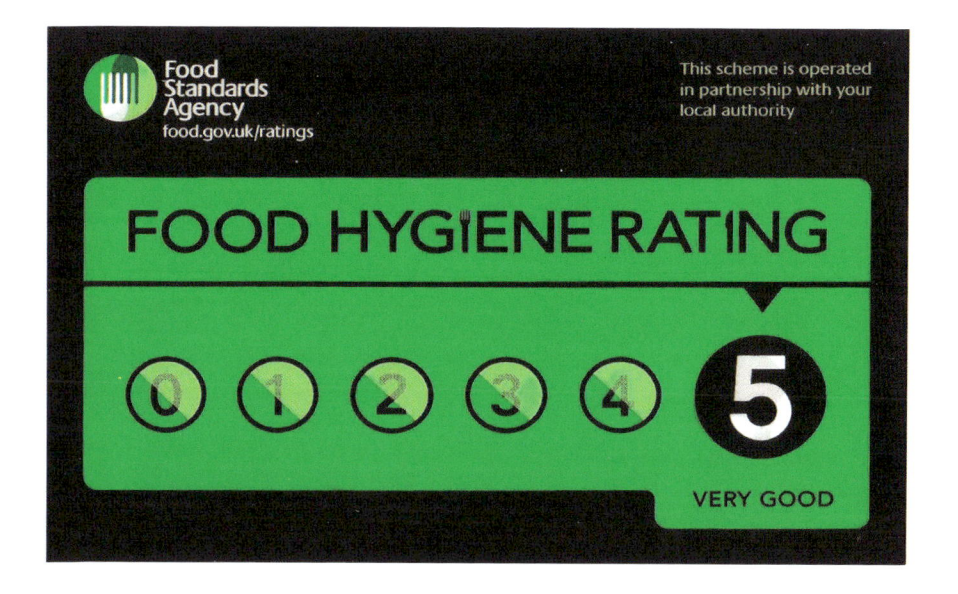

This book is protected under the copywrite laws. Any reproductions or other unauthorised use of the material herein is prohibited without the express written permission of the author.

Copyright © by Jennifer King
All rights reserved

ISBN: 9798734183748

Disclaimer

Although the author and publisher have made every effort to ensure that the information in this book was correct at the time of publication, the author and publisher do not assume and hereby disclaim any liability to any party for any loss, damage or disruption from use or misuse of the information provided in this book.

CONTENTS

DISCLAIMER   2

INTRODUCTION   4

1. DIFFERENT TYPES OF CARE HOMES   6

2. DOMICILIARY CARE (ALSO KNOWN AS HOMECARE)   7

3. THE HEALTH REGULATOR   8

4. WHO MAY NEED CARE?   10

5. UNDERSTANDING THE DIFFERENT TYPES OF DEMENTIA   11

6. UNDERSTANDING COMMON HEALTH CONDITIONS   14

7. THINGS TO CONSIDER WHEN CHOOSING CARE   15

8. THINGS TO CHECK WHEN VISITING A CARE HOME   21

9. FUNDING STREAMS   23

10. NHS HEALTH FUNDING   23

11. LOCAL AUTHORITY FUNDING   25

12. UNDERSTANDING FINANCIAL ASSESSMENTS/ MEANS TESTING   26

13. ALTERNATIVE OPTIONS TO SELLING YOUR HOME SHOULD YOU NOT QUALIFY FOR FUNDING   27

14. MENTAL CAPACITY/POWER OF ATTORNEY   28

15. INDEPENDENT ADVOCACY   28

16. OTHER IMPORTANT INFORMATION   29

17. RECAP ON COMMONLY BELIEVED MYTHS   30

        FINAL THOUGHTS   31

Introduction

Choosing care in later years for yourself or a loved one is difficult at the best of times. However, there are many options available to you and I will guide you through these at this worrying time. From initial checks (such as food hygiene ratings), to inspection reports and spot checks, you will be empowered to quality check and ensure that ongoing care also continues. Daunting as it seems, once you have an understanding, things are quite straightforward and I will clarify some commonly believed myths which will surprise you.

Having worked as a care home inspector and as a health care professional, I know what is required to make decisions on care and funding. If eligible, some funding is not means tested (you could be a millionaire and it would not matter) and would therefore be free with nothing to pay back ever! Do not assume that someone will be kind enough to tell you your full entitlement, they will not. It is left to you to find out whether you are getting your full entitlement and to also ask for it. Furthermore, you will be encouraged to obtain a copy of the decision-making assessment and consider an appeal, should any decision be declined. The book is a valuable source of information and almost certainly not welcomed by both the Local Authorities and health (NHS) for sharing the tools they use for making funding decisions.

I will tell you how means testing works for finance and the things which are disregarded for means testing.

Whilst worked in health, I saw many people worrying about choosing care for their loved ones. Most people do not have any idea on where to start (and why would they). I found myself explaining time and time again, the routes on offer, most of which is not freely given to people who should otherwise obtain funding rightfully due to them. I found this unfair and unjust. I think most people who paid their taxes through their whole life, believe that this care is already paid for; it should be this way but sadly it is not. When people are in the position of finding care, the realisation of just what needs to be done, can be quite challenging. The thought of a loved one no longer being able to care for themselves is traumatic enough, let alone the things you have to put in place.

The cost of care is continually rising. People are living much longer, which is fantastic and the need to support the elderly is increasing. This of course places pressures on services which has to be taken into account, hence the reason why funding is getting more difficult to obtain. With stricter guidelines in place, there is however, help out there and a lot of good care is provided.

The average care home costs anywhere between £800 - £1200 per week, so it is important to get things in place and this includes funding, which of course plays a part.

On a very positive note, some people even choose to go into care homes to be with other people. Some care homes are so well set up they even have private flats for people to live in. It is a bit like supported living but in reality, it is like living in a hotel. I've spoken to many people who just love being in this type of set-up and feel very safe too.

Whatever your reasons for having care, most challenges will be covered in this book.

1. Different Types of Care Homes

When people think of care, they think of 'Care Homes' in general. However, it is important to know the difference between care homes as there are two types which are very different dependent on needs.

Residential Homes - a residential home does not require a nurse to be on site. Most of the care is carried out by carers. These homes usually attract residents with lower needs than that of a nursing home. However, District Nurses may still attend site for dressings etc.

Nursing Homes - a nursing home, as the name suggests, has a nurse on site. There has to be at least one registered nurse at site (see Section 16 to check a nurse's registration and fitness to practice). A nursing home usually attracts but not always, people with higher needs, such as tracheostomy residents etc. These residents need a higher level of care, hence a nurse needs to be on hand 24/7. Although the nurse will not always do all tasks herself/himself, they will be at least responsible for clinical events on site. A nursing home, may still have residential residents at the home and some of these residents may have District Nursing attending site frequently to undertake certain tasks such as changing dressings etc. Although the nurse in a nursing home has overall clinical responsibility, she/he generally carries out nursing tasks for 'nurse funded' residents.

Supported living - these services offer extra care for people to live in. this can be by living in a self-contained bungalow or flat and assistance can be called upon 24/7. This type of care is usually for those that do not need have high levels of care.

2. Domiciliary Care (also known as Homecare)

Many people refer to this as Homecare but it is known in the UK as Domiciliary care. There are many providers giving service on behalf of either the Local Authority, National Health Service or privately.

The care itself works in the same way as in a **residential home** but the carers or district nurses attend the person's home. Often, there will be a key safe on the wall of the person's home for the carer or district nurse to gain access for anyone who is bed-bound. If you have a loved one who is bed-bound, then I would suggest removing any valuables from the property, I have seen too often that things tend to go missing. There have been many safeguarding incidents I have been involved in alleging that carers have stolen money or valuables.

When choosing a provider of this service, word of mouth or speaking to the Local Authority is a starting point. The Local Authorities usually have a list of providers they use and they will also inspect these services too. Most sections of this book are also relevant for domiciliary care.

Make sure that you claim for all the benefits you're entitled to. Things like Attendance Allowance is a benefit for people over state pension age who need extra help to stay independent at home, due to an illness or disability. Additionally, if you are under state pension age, you could be eligible for a personal independence payment instead. A carer could be eligible for a carer's allowance also.

Funding is covered in great depth, further in the book.

3. The Health Regulator

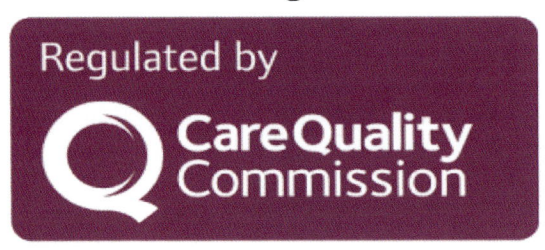

The Care Quality Commission (CQC) is the independent regulator of all health and social care services in England, be it for NHS settings, private hospitals, dentists, domiciliary care etc. Inspection reports can be found on their website for you to view at any time. The Care Quality Commission should inspect services every 2-3 years if there are no known concerns and more often if there are concerns. The inspection team ideally should have a clinician but often do not. There is usually a small team consisting of Inspectors, Experts-by experience, Independent Assessors or any other person from a quality perspective. For care homes, the provider must display their CQC rating in areas for all to see. They are usually found as you enter the care home and it also should be visible on their website. Domiciliary care providers must display their CQC rating at the office address. Some providers I have found have not displayed their rating if they have a poor rating. The CQC can impose sanctions and put a provider into special measures if they are dissatisfied by the level of care provided. Care homes and domiciliary providers have to report certain events to the CQC, for example, all deaths in care homes are notifiable to the CQC as are certain safeguarding issues, such as serious pressure ulcers. You can contact the CQC should you have concerns

England - Care Quality Commission

Wales - Care Inspectorate Wales

Scotland - Care Inspectorate

The CQC assesses areas of: Safety, Effective, Caring, Responsive and Well-led with the ratings shown below. An Overall rating from each of these areas is then given.

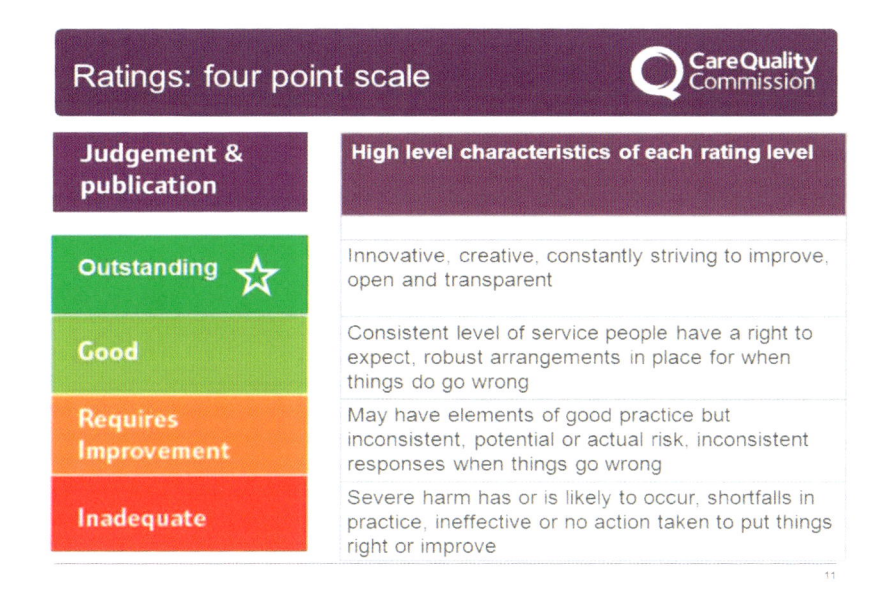

Ratings: four point scale — CareQuality Commission

Judgement & publication	High level characteristics of each rating level
Outstanding ☆	Innovative, creative, constantly striving to improve, open and transparent
Good	Consistent level of service people have a right to expect, robust arrangements in place for when things do go wrong
Requires Improvement	May have elements of good practice but inconsistent, potential or actual risk, inconsistent responses when things go wrong
Inadequate	Severe harm has or is likely to occur, shortfalls in practice, ineffective or no action taken to put things right or improve

Previous reports can also be viewed. **Take note**, some providers, particularly domiciliary care providers change their company name when they receive a poor rating. However, the CQC website can often reveal this as a link to a previous company name so do your homework. A 'Good' rating in all areas will look something like this

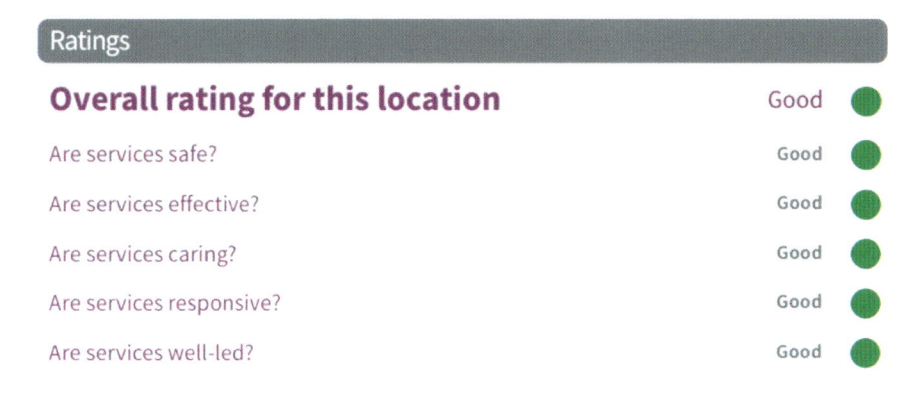

Ratings

Overall rating for this location — Good

Are services safe?	Good
Are services effective?	Good
Are services caring?	Good
Are services responsive?	Good
Are services well-led?	Good

4. Who may need care?

It is difficult to believe that we all may need some sort of care. I see this as a plus, especially in later years as it serves as a reminder that someone is living a long life. Although there are some babies, children and young adults who sadly need care due to brain damage etc, we are going to look at elderly care.

As we get older, everything slows down but this does not mean our lives cannot be fulfilling. People needing care may be for reasons such as:

. Physical health needs mean they can no longer look after themselves. Examples of this could be that someone continues to fall in their home. This can be obviously dangerous, especially for those living alone. The risk of someone falling increases significantly as we reach our later years. Another example is people who are on end-of-life care. A lot of people think that Hospices and Hospitals are the right place but these are not always the right place for everyone. If someone can be nursed in their own home, then this can be a viable option and is often the choice of the person involved.

. Personal care, washing and bathing

. Cooking and cleaning (in own home)

. Dementia (see Section 5)

. An increase in the number of home visits a day by district nurses, doctors etc may suggest care could be considered.

. Choice - lots of people take this choice as they do not like living alone or family do not live nearby.

5. Understanding the different types of Dementia

One of the main reasons why people go into a care home is because of dementia. Most people get confused with the different names but it is important to know that they all fall under the generic name of **'Dementia'**. This section explains the most common types.

Dementia is the generic term used for a range of symptoms which includes memory loss, difficulty with speaking and making decisions. Changes begin as minor but over time will start to affect a person's daily life and their mood and behaviour is likely to alter too. Dementia occurs when the brain is damaged by diseases such as Alzheimer's disease. Dementia and Alzheimer's disease are not separate diseases, they fall under the generic term of Dementia. The common types of Dementia are:

(a) Alzheimer's disease
Named after the doctor who invented the disease, Alois Alzheimer. Alzheimer's disease is **the most common** type of dementia.

Why does this happen? The brain is made up of billions of nerve cells connected to each other. When these connections are lost; the disease can occur. Furthermore, proteins build up and form *plaques* and *tangles*. Nerve cells die causing tissue to be lost. Additionally, the chemicals which send signals between cells are greatly reduced for people with Alzheimer's disease.

Can anything be done? There are drugs available which may help with some of the conditions. There is lots of research on keeping the mind active taking place, which may or may not help to reduce symptoms of this disease. It is important to know however, that this disease usually worsens over time. It is estimated that there are more than 500,000 people in the United Kingdom diagnosed with dementia, caused by Alzheimer's disease and it is thought that these figures will only rise.

(b) Alzheimer's disease with Lewy bodies
Named after a German Neurologist, Lewy noticed that there were abnormal deposits of protein that would disrupt the brain's normal functioning in people that had Parkinson's disease. These abnormal deposits are known as Lewy bodies. Although it is not fully known what causes Lewy bodies or how they contribute to dementia, they do seem to appear to be linked to two factors:
1. low levels of acetylcholine and dopamine, both of which carry messages between nerve cells.
2. loss of the connections between the nerve cells which then die.

Lewy bodies at the base of the brain usually affects movement and is the main feature in Parkinson's disease.

Lewy bodies found in the outer layers of the brain are usually linked with mental abilities.

It is also possible for people to have problems with both their movement and mental abilities.

(c) Vascular dementia
This is the **second most common** type of dementia in people over the age of 65. Vascular dementia is caused by problems with blood circulation to the brain. Examples of this are:
. Blocked arteries
. Transient Ischaemic Attacks (TIAs - a mini stroke)
. Stroke - larger type stroke

The drugs used for Alzheimer's are not usually beneficial for those who have vascular dementia. However, if this type of dementia is caused by heart disease, diabetes or stroke, a change of lifestyle and medication can prevent the disease from progressing.

(d) Alcohol related dementia
This type of dementia is, as the name suggests, brain damage related to alcohol. Someone suffering from this type of dementia will have problems with memory loss, daily tasks

and living. The excessive drinking will have caused damage to the brain. However, if the excessive drinking is stopped and there is a change in lifestyle, there can be a degree of partial recovery.

(e) Frontotemporal dementia
Less common, especially in people over the age of 65. It is caused by the death of nerve cells in the frontal and temporal parts of the brain. It is progressive and affects behaviour and personality.

(f) Huntington's disease
This disease is inherited and usually begins to affect people aged 30-50. There is no cure and the disease will progressively get worse. Signs include; memory lapses, stumbling, involuntary movements of the body etc.

(g) Parkinson's Disease Dementia
Someone with Parkinson's disease has a high risk of developing dementia (Parkinson's disease dementia) as their conditions worsens.

Be mindful also, that a person can have a mixture of dementia. An Example being someone with Alzheimer's disease and Vascular dementia. This type of **Mixed dementia** is common in people that are over 75 years of age.

Dementia is one of the main reasons why people go into care. Sometimes it is for their own safety as often, dementia sufferers tend to wander and get themselves lost or even worse. Consideration needs to be given to people with dementia living in their own homes too. Often things like changing the gas cooker to an electric oven can reduce potential problems. Of all the diseases out there, dementia is one of the hardest to manage by family members and an extremely popular reason for considering care for a loved one.

6. Understanding Common Health Conditions

This section will deal with a few common reasons why people are unable to look after themselves.

Section 5 has covered Dementia in great detail as it is one of the main reasons people need care. The danger that someone can be in with dementia should never be underestimated.

Falls is another reason why someone may need care because as we age, our risk of falls increases significantly. Add this to the fact that bones get more brittle as we age, the risk of injury, serious and permanent injury increases dramatically.

Pressure ulcer - albeit serious ones, could be a reason for needing care.

Acquired brain injuries - these range from people having aneurysms, injuries following accidents such as car accidents, stokes etc.

Neglect is a reason why the elderly go into care or due to abuse (sadly at times by immediate family members).

An illness which means that someone cannot look after themselves physically, mentally or both.

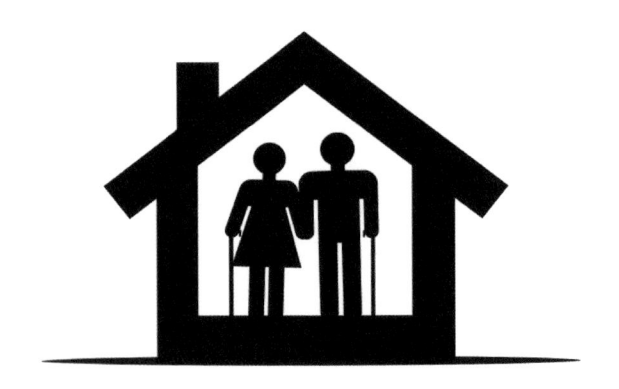

7. Things to consider when choosing care

Far be it for anyone to tell you what is important for you or a loved one but I have included some things which you may or may not wish to consider.

I have inspected many care homes, both nursing and residential, as well as domiciliary providers. There are large companies with infrastructures in place for governance etc. There are also small care providers privately run as a small family business. It is unfair to say which is the best as ultimately, it is down to the individual care provider. Larger companies are accused of putting profit first but they also have deep pockets, whereby smaller individual providers are sometimes criticized for 'penny pinching'. As I say, it is all really down to the provider and following some guidelines, will put you in the best position to choose the right care. I have seen the best and worst of care and cannot tell you whether I think the larger companies are better than the smaller companies. Ultimately, the manager and clinical leads are key in care. A good manager will ensure standards are high, things like nail polish and jewellery is not worn by staff and that staff are bare below the elbow (as they should be). Some basic standards say a lot and you will usually pick up a sense if something is not right. This section will give you some pointers to help you make an informed decision. Work out what is important for you and here are some things which I think are important for you to make an informed choice.

This section can help you also find the best domiciliary care for you/ a loved one. Not all will be applicable for domiciliary care but a lot will be.

. **Food/Nutrition** - food and drink is very important and although as we age, we eat less, for many elderly people, they still enjoy food and want a varied diet. Care homes (nursing and residential) should be able to show you their menus. Often, these menus have a 4 week rolling rota for meals and some homes will alter these menus for summer and winter. Check whether residents would be able to deviate from the menu or have at least a snack should they become hungry between meals or at night. Drinks should also be plentiful. Again, as we age, fluids are still important and play a part in reducing pressure ulcers. You may wish to see whether guests can stay for meals and if so, whether there is a charge.

Food hygiene ratings - most providers making or serving food, must both have and display a food hygiene rating. These are rated by the Local Authority and range from 0 (worst) to the best score of 5. I have sadly witnessed a home with a 0 rating. The home was ordered to close the kitchen due to a rat infestation and poor storage of food. As it is not feasible to just close a care home, as a lot of things needs to be considered before moving people, the home was instructed to have food brought in. Thankfully, the home made the necessary improvements and then received a new rating of 4. It is not just care homes which have ratings, places which serve food - takeaways, restaurants, pubs etc all legally have to display their ratings. If they do not, ask to see the rating. These ratings are usually done every 2-3 years, so a low rating is likely to stay with the provider for some time unless there are exceptional cases, such as the one I have mentioned with the 0 rating. When you are next out at a restaurant, look out for these signs. England, Northern Ireland and Wales have a similar system, Scotland has a slightly different way of rating.

Food Hygiene – England, Northern Ireland and Wales

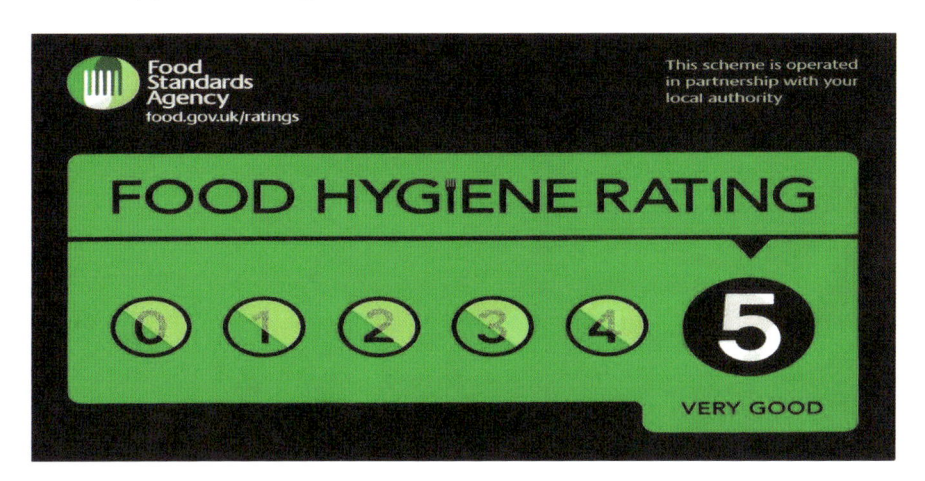

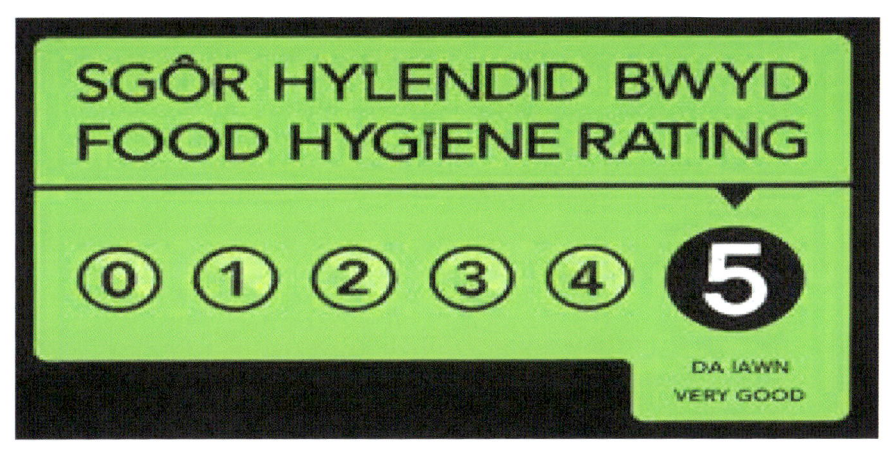

Total score	0 - 15	20	25 - 30	35 - 40	45 - 50	> 50
Maximum scoring factor	No score greater than 5	No score greater than 10	No score greater than 10	No score greater than 15	No score greater than 20	-
Rating	5 (top)	4	3	2	1	0 (bottom)
Hygiene standards	Very good	Good	Generally satisfactory	Improvement necessary	Major improvement necessary	Urgent improvement necessary

Food Hygiene rating - England and Wales

Food Hygiene Rating	Description
⓪①②③④**⑤** Very good	Very Good
⓪①②③**④**⑤ Good	Good
⓪①②**③**④⑤ Generally satisfactory	Generally Satisfactory
⓪①**②**③④⑤ Improvement necessary	Improvement Necessary
⓪**①**②③④⑤ Major improvement necessary	Major Improvement Necessary
⓪①②③④⑤ Urgent improvement necessary	Urgent Improvement Necessary

Scotland

Scotland has a slightly different system. Inspections are graded by the Local Authority but the ratings are usually: **Pass** or **Improvement Required**.

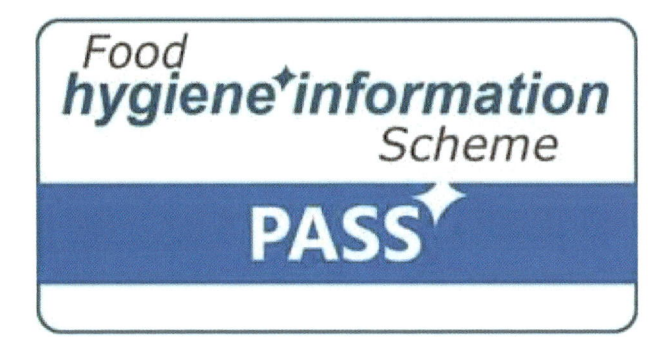

Location - is it important for the care home to be close to where loved ones are? Make a list of care homes nearby and look at the CQC ratings. You may also have recommendations from people you know. This is a valuable resource.

Places of Worship/ Religion - places of worship may be important to be close by, or perhaps the home offers these services to come to site such as Sunday Services, Priests etc.

Pets - you may have a pet and many care homes allow pets to either live at the home or have no issue if a pet visits the home.

Garden - a garden or outside space may be important.

Visiting times/restrictions - check whether you can visit at any time. Some care homes have protected mealtimes for residents. Also see whether there are any restrictions on children visiting. See also comments in Section 7 on whether guests can stay for meals.

Staff training - you may not think that this is important but you need to know whether staff are trained adequately and that this is ongoing. Never be afraid to ask to see the Training Matrix, which will perhaps shock some care managers. Training should include at the very least:
. Fire safety
. Medicines Management
. Moving and handling
. Infection prevention and control
. Pressure ulcer - also known as tissue viability
. Basic life support/first aid
. Equality and diversity
. Safeguarding
. Food hygiene

The better homes will invest in their staff and have additional training available. I would expect the compliance for training to be at least 90%. If not, ask the manager how this is being addressed or find another care home.

Staff ratios and agency usage - this was something which I frequently criticised when inspecting a care home. Staff costs will always be the highest cost for any business, however, not having enough staff is both dangerous and irresponsible. Ask to see rotas, to include overnight. There is no exact science on numbers as this depends whether the home has high levels of dementia, if the home has different floors etc. the CQC reports will also usually comment on staffing.

Same sex carers - this may or may not be important to you.

Regular meetings - are there meetings for both residents and relatives? Ask to see the recent minutes etc. Although, issues should not wait until a meeting takes place, the better homes will have monthly meetings and drop in sessions/coffee mornings.

Surveys - ask to see the last survey for residents and relatives/friends. Surveys should be conducted at least annually, with actions for any negative feedback being addressed. You should see actions like 'you said, we did'.

Waiting list notice period - you should know whether there is a waiting list. If there is, this reflects the home is likely to be a good home. Also, ensure you know what the minimum notice period is, should you wish to give notice.

ACTIVITIES COORDINATORS - I cannot stress to you just how important this is. A home with nothing to do other than watch television, is a home you should steer clear from. There should be at least 1 full time activities co-ordinator working during the days. The better homes will have cover at weekends. Things like games, quizzes, animals visiting, entertainers, movie days, outings offsite to the beach etc. There may be some additional charges for trips out of the home but these are usually minimal. A home with nobody to do this essential role, is not worth considering in my view.

Appointments (doctors, dentists, opticians) - just because someone is at a care home, they should still have these appointments. The gold standard would be that a doctor visits weekly but not all care homes will be able to offer this. If possible, opt for a home which is proactive with the local GP surgeries. Someone in a care home should also have, at the minimum, an annual medication review by their doctor. Additionally, dental and optician appointments are equally important, although these may have to be done off site.

Complaints - ask to see the complaints policy, ALL care homes and domiciliary providers should have one.

English not the first language - this may be important to you. Some care providers have carers who can interpret and if your loved one has little or poor English, you may need to consider this.

Assessment - unless you/your loved one is self-funding the placement at the home, a needs assessment will also need to be done – see Sections 9-12 (inclusive).

8. Things to check when visiting a care home

One thing I would always advocate, is to turn up unannounced during the day but check that there are vacancies beforehand. If the care home is worth considering, you should be welcomed and shown around, meeting both the manager and staff. The care home manager may not appreciate it but you need to see the care home as it really is. Things like having to wait outside for 10 minutes before someone lets you in will certainly annoy you if it becomes a regular thing. To be fair though, I would avoid lunch times as staff are very busy, so turn up mid-morning or mid-afternoon.

As well as looking at the CQC Report, Food Hygiene rating and the things in Section 7, there are some things you should take note of whilst visiting.

- Are the buildings and grounds maintained?
- Ask to see a room and see whether it is what you want and is comfortable. Consider whether a personal bathroom in the room is important or whether sharing facilities is acceptable.
- Does the home smell? I've been to too many care homes where this is the case. It is not always the carpeted care homes either, even the ones with hard flooring can often smell of stale urine etc.
- If the needs of care change, can the home cope with this? Often nursing homes are well equipped but consider that your loved one may need to move care home, which is far from ideal.
- Look at the food menus, inspect the kitchens.
- Can personal furniture be taken to the care home to make the room more personal?
- Ask to see policies and procedures and the training matrix
- Speak to any visitors and staff at the home to try and gauge their feelings about the home
- Ask to see what is included in the home's insurance
- Is there a tie-in period to stay at the home?
- Speak to the Activities Co-ordinator to see if there is a plan of activities and ask to see photographs of any activities which have taken place.
- Look to see whether there are pull cords in the room (usually located next to where the bed is and in bathrooms too).

9. Funding Streams

The next few sections are about funding. The first thing to note is that funding can come from:
. Health (NHS)
. Local Authority
. Joint funded - which is funded by both health and the local authority.

Funding applies for both care homes and domiciliary care (care at home). Also note, that funding is becoming more and more tight with both the local authorities and health tightening their belts. Even if you are thinking of funding the care yourself, please check first whether you are eligible for some or all funding.

10. Health (NHS) Funding

Health Funding is broken down into two main categories, following an assessment of needs:

(1) NHS Continuing Health Care (CHC) - this funding is generally for people who have high needs. If you are eligible for what is known as full CHC funding, you will not be means tested. Basically, if you are a millionaire, you will not need to pay anything back, ever. Take into account though, that there will be (or should be) an annual review of funding, so it can be withdrawn by another assessment in future.
To obtain this funding, a person must have a **Primary** health need. Do not think that having dementia qualifies, it often does not. A Checklist is done first and you can request this at any time (all assessments are free). The checklist will ascertain whether a full assessment is needed and you can ask for this at any time (now and in the future). The checklist should be done within 14 days, although this timescale usually slips. For a full assessment, an assessor, who is usually a nurse, will

use a Decision Support Tool. Take note of the decision and try and be present (with the elderly person's permission) when these assessments are done. Believe me, some nurses will say at assessment that you are highly likely to get funding, only for the opposite be reflected in a letter. Note the name of the nurse and which organisation she/he works for. Very important, you **MUST** obtain a copy of the assessment. Whatever excuse you are given, keep asking and if necessary, ask the person being assessed, to request a copy of their assessment as this cannot be refused.

If you feel that the decision is unjust, there is an appeals process, so ask for the appeals procedure.

Domains - assessors will look at domains of: Behaviour, Cognition, Mobility, Breathing, Nutrition, Continence, Medication, Altered states of consciousness, Tissue viability, Psychological needs, Communication and Other significant care needs. If assessed as 'Severe' in two or more domains then you are likely to be eligible for this funding (gradings are Low, Moderate, High or Severe).

If **one 'Priority'** is found in certain domains, then you are likely to be eligible for this funding.

Priority grading examples would be for:
. Someone who is unable to breathe independently and requiring ventilation
. Challenging behaviour which is severe frequent and/or is unpredictable.
. Having a drug regime requiring daily monitoring by a registered nurse to control symptom and pain management.
. Altered states of consciousness occurring on most days, which results in severe risk of harm.

IMPORTANT - hospitals are well known for getting people out of hospital as soon as possible. You/your loved one may be placed at a care home on what is known as a 'Fast Track'. This means you will not have to pay for the first 12 weeks until a review has been done. People sometimes fall into the trap of believing that this care is therefore free on full CHC funding, even after the 12 weeks. I have

known assessments to be done and an elderly person sadly has had to move out of the care home to a less expensive care home due to being unable to meet the costs after review. Fast Track is also sometimes used for an end of life package of care.

(2) Funded Nursing Care (FNC) - this is a flat rate that the NHS pays to a care home or domiciliary provider towards their care. Note, this payment is approximately £200 per week. The elderly person would (as FNC suggests) need to require nursing care in order to qualify.

11. Local Authority Funding

This funding is available in a similar manner to that of health. A needs test, which is free, would be needed to establish the level of care needed. Dependent on savings, there may be full, partial or no funding available. Following an assessment, if the Local Authority deem you to need a care home (usually residential), a financial (also known as social care) assessment will take place. To give you an approximate idea; if you have **savings** and **assets** of:
. Less than £14,000 - you may qualify for full support but may still have to contribute from any income received
. £14,000 - £24,000 - you may qualify for partial payment
. Over £24,000 - you will be deemed to be a self-funder and likely to have to pay for care yourself

12. Understanding financial assessments/ means testing

It is important that you understand how means testing (also known as financial assessments) is done and how assessments are carried out. Things like savings, property, pensions, investments and some benefits will be taken into account for means testing. As well as the approximate figures from savings and assets, there are some important things that you need to know about if you/a loved one needs to go into a care home. Many people are terrified that they will have to sell their home should they need care but take note:

DISREGARDED = it will not be counted

If you own your home and you live there alone, it is likely that this would be included as part of your capital for purposes of means testing for a care home. **VERY IMPORTANT - if your:**
. **Spouse**
. **Partner**
. **Children under the age of 16 (that are your children)**
. **Relative aged 60 or over**
. **Disabled relative**

would continue to live in your home, your home will be **'disregarded'** for any financial assessment.

Your home will also not be included in a financial assessment if you receive care and support at home **(domiciliary care)**, again, it will be **'disregarded'**.

Many people are relieved to know this and this is possibly one of the greatest pieces of knowledge you need to know regarding funding. When I have told people this, they were always astonished.

If, for any reason, your home is to be included in your means test, they must also take joint ownership into consideration and only look at your share. Additionally, the Local Authority usually ignores it for the first 12 weeks of your care. Spend this time wisely to decide if you are going to sell your home or opt for a deferred payment (see Section 13).

13. Alternative options to selling your home should you not qualify for funding

I will start this section by the temptation of many, to consider giving away a property to children or relatives. This can be very risky as it is counted as a 'deprivation of assets'. This could mean that you may still have to pay the same level of care fees as you would if you still had your home. Additionally, gambling, giving money away, spending in an unusual way, using savings for buying jewellery, cars etc would count too. Of course, if you did any of this when you were fit and healthy, this would not be counted as deprivation of assets.

Renting property - some people rent their property to help pay for fees and this could be an excellent option for you to consider.

Deferred payment agreement - this is a viable option to delay selling a home to pay for care. This works by having a legal agreement with your Local Authority (usually involving a legal charge on your property with HM Land Registry). The condition of this agreement is that the fees owed would be paid at a later date (usually on death), when the costs would be paid through your estate. Deferred payment agreements are also sometimes utilised as a bridging loan to allow time for the sale of a property.

The most common reason for someone to have a deferred payment agreement is when savings and assets (apart from the home) are low but the value of their home is taking them over the threshold for paying for care.

However, please always remember the very important 'disregarded' information in Section 12.

14. Mental Capacity/ Power of Attorney

The capacity of someone is very important to understand, you will often hear it in the context of MCA (Mental Capacity Act). Capacity assessments are made if there is a concern that someone may lack capacity. In general, capacity is assumed but if there is any doubt, then a 'capacity assessment' should be carried out. A person can have capacity for some decisions but not others and this is where relatives/friends come in. You may be aware of a Lasting Power of Attorney; however, did you know that there are separate ones for health and finance? One person may have power of attorney for health and another person could have it for finance. Ideally, this should be arranged before anyone loses their capacity. If there are no relatives or friends, then it is up to clinicians to make 'Best Interest' decisions on their behalf. At times, if families are quarrelling, the decision would fall to the Court to decide and if a decision cannot be made, a solicitor for example may be appointed to have the Lasting Power of Attorney.
It is important in the case of decision making that you know where you stand, as you cannot make decisions for people who have not appointed you to do so. Similarly, if a person has capacity and can therefore make their own decisions, you cannot overrule these in the same way that someone else cannot do so for you.

15. Independent Advocacy

For anyone struggling to make decisions about care and has no one to help with this, they have a right to an Independent Advocate. Do not worry about this as there are lots of people who can help. To obtain further details, contact your Local Authority and ask for one of these advocates.

16. Other important information

. Check a Nurse's registration to practice - In the UK, there is a register which nurses have to be registered on. It is the Nursing and Midwifery Council (NMC) www.nmc.org.uk and you can access this online and free of charge. You do not need their registration number and can search by name. This would usually apply for Nursing homes but also any nurses which may be caring for you or a loved one. All nurses have to re-register annually. Any fitness to practice (current or past) will be shown for you to see. You can also report any urgent concerns to the NMC. Similarly, there is the medical register for Doctors. The General Medical Council (GMC), is a list of doctors in the United Kingdom, showing their registration status, training and other useful information. Again, it is free at www.gmc-uk.org or (www.gdc-uk.org for dentists).

. Obvious signs of poor care - sadly, I have seen all too often tell-tale signs of poor care. For example, you may see excrement on walls and under the fingernails of people with dementia. Clearly, they are not to blame but it also needs to be managed properly. It is an easy way for you to note poor care. Nails should be kept clean and if you see this (or anything similar), you need to question it, as this is basic hygiene, what else is being ignored?

. Participation of care - you should participate in any care that you can (if you are entitled to). This includes care plans, attending meetings and regularly speaking to the managers and staff of the care home or domiciliary care company.

. Whistleblowing and Safeguarding concerns - some people are reluctant to complain, as they are then leaving their loved one to be looked after by the very same people. There really comes a point when you may have to report things to either the Local Authority, CQC or even the Police. You know what is right and wrong and so do care staff, so if it feels wrong, it probably is.

17. Recap on commonly believed myths

You have taken in a lot of information and I hope you retain this book as a guide and to recap on. I feel that perhaps the most commonly believed myth, relates to means testing and having to sell a home. I therefore have chosen to repeat some information below from Section 12, as a reminder for both care homes and domiciliary care.

Property, pensions, investments and some benefits will be taken into account for means testing. There are some important things that you need to know about if you/a loved one needs to go into a care home or have domiciliary care. Many people are terrified that they will have to sell their home should they need care, take note:

DISREGARDED = it will not be counted

If you own your home and you live there alone, it is likely that this would be included as part of your capital for purposes of means testing for a care home. **VERY IMPORTANT – If your:**
. **Spouse**
. **Partner**
. **Children under the age of 16 (that are your children)**
. **Relative aged 60 or over**
. **Disabled relative**
would continue to live in your home, your home will be **'disregarded'** for any financial assessment.

Your home will also not be included in a financial assessment if you receive care and support at home **(domiciliary care)**, again, it will be **'disregarded'**.

Final Thoughts

This is a daunting time for all but hopefully this book has given you some important advice on how to find care and ensure quality standards are maintained. The myths people have on funding is also major feedback I receive, along with the relief, once understood that it is not a given to sell a property to fund care.

Take this book with you when sourcing care, write in pencil as you go through things you have checked on.

Good luck with everything and thanks for reading.

Jennifer

Printed in Great Britain
by Amazon